HOW TO RESTORE YOUR VISION

THROUGH SCIENTIFICALLY PROVEN EYE EXERCISES

Here we'll discuss specific eye problems, their causes and the recommended eye exercises that will help to diminish or cure them, then in the next section, we'll go into detail regarding the eye exercises and how you can do them at home without interrupting your daily activities.

Listed below are the various eye problems and the recommended eye exercises to diminish or cure them.

Presbyopia & Hyperopia (Farsightedness)

Cause:

Presbyopia is an eye condition where the lens of your eye loses its flexibility. This loss of flexibility makes it difficult to focus on close objects. Presbyopia is similar to Hyperopia, but is an age related eye condition that occurs around age 40, where the aging of the eye deteriorates the lens. Hyperopia (or Farsightedness) is an eye condition where distant objects appear clear, but close objects appear blurred. Hyperopia occurs when your eyeball is too short, or the cornea has too little curvature (opposite of Myopia). Too little curvature causes light entering the eye to not focus correctly on the retina.

Exercises:

The goal of this exercise routine is to increase the nutrient flow in the eye and maximize flexibility of the inner lens. If you have Presbyopia or Hyperopia, you will benefit from the exercise routine below:

Exercise Routine	Duration: 30 mins.
Palming	3 minutes
Eye Rolls	2 minute
Clock Rotations	4 minute
Squeeze Blinking	1 minute
Pumping	2 minutes
Tromboning	2 minutes
Acupressure 4	5 minutes
Blur Zoning	3 minutes
Shifting	3 minutes
Hydrotherapy	5 minutes

Myopia (Nearsightedness)

Cause:

Myopia (or nearsightedness) is an eye condition where objects up close appear clear, but objects farther away appear blurred. This is caused when the eyeball or cornea is too long or has too much of a curvature. This over curvature causes light entering the eye to be unfocused on the retina which sends the blurred vision to the brain through the optic nerve. Myopia can be caused by visual stress of doing too much work associated with close range vision, such as reading, or computer work. However adult myopia is usually caused by visual stress, as well as health conditions, such as diabetes.

Exercises:

If you have Myopia (or nearsightedness), use the exercise routine below. On top of these exercises it is important to break any habits of reading up close, such as reading books, newspapers and using computers or laptops. Going outside and using your long-range vision is key. Playing certain long-range games such as golf, Frisbee, tennis or bowling could help cure your Myopia.

Exercise Routine	Duration: 25 mins.
Palming	3 minutes
Pumping	2 minutes
Blur Zoning	3 minutes
Acupressure 4	5 minutes
Eye Rolls	2 minutes
Squeeze Blinking	2 minutes
Clock Rotations	3 minutes
Hydrotherapy	5 minutes

Astigmatism

Cause:

Astigmatism is an eye condition that causes blurred vision at any distance. This is caused by an irregular shaped cornea or irregular curvature of the lens. Most people with Astigmatism have bad posture, and their head usually tilts towards a side. This causes the extraocular muscles of the eye to work overtime, by adjusting to the new vision which is slightly tilted.

Exercises:

This exercise routine is specifically designed for people with Astigmatism. You may find your eyes become sore after the exercises. If this occurs, follow up with the Eyestrain exercise routine to sooth your sore eyes. Along with the exercises it's important to correct the posture of your neck. To do this, place sticky notes angled in the opposite direction of your head tilt in various places around your home – your bathroom mirror, near the kitchen sink, on the pantry, on the wall near the bed, etc. This will force you to tilt your head in the opposite direction every time you see the tilted sticky notes. Eventually your posture will improve automatically.

Exercise Routine	Duration: 30 mins.
Palming	3 minutes
Eye Rolls	2 minute
Clock Rotations	3 minute
Acupressure 1	2 minutes
Eye Rolls	2 minute
Clock Rotations	3 minute
Acupressure 2	2 minutes
Eye Rolls	2 minute
Clock Rotations	3 minute
Acupressure 3	2 minutes
Squeeze Blinking	2 minute
Slow Blinking	1 minute
Hydrotherapy	3 minutes

Amblyopia & Strabismus (Lazy Eye & Crossed Eyes)

Cause:

Amblyopia (or Lazy Eye) is the lack of development or loss of central vision in one eye. This is usually unrelated to any health problem and is not corrected using lenses. Amblyopia is caused by failure to use both eyes together. You will notice a lazy eye, by one eye always looking in a different direction compared to the good eye. Amblyopia is often associated with Strabismus (Crossed Eyes) which is an eye condition where both eyes do not look in the same direction at the same time. Strabismus is usually caused by poor extraocular muscles of the eye. Although you can usually notice a person with Amblyopia or Strabismus, it can be brought on by tired or strained eyes, excessive reading or computer work, or when the person is fighting an illness like a cold or flu.

Exercises:

If you have a Lazy Eye or are Crossed Eyed, an eye patch over the dominate eye, usually the non-lazy eye, for several hours a day will help the weaker eye to develop. How to determine your dominate eye:

- Extend both your hands in front of your body, and create a small triangle by overlapping your thumbs and overlapping your fingers to the first knuckle.
- With both eyes open, look through the triangle and center an object in the middle – such as a doorknob (something small enough to fit into the triangle).
- Close your LEFT eye only – if the object remains in the triangle you are RIGHT eye dominate.
- Close your RIGHT eye only – if the object remains in the triangle you are LEFT eye dominate.

Once the weaker eye is working better, continue with the Myopia and Presbyopia/Hyperopia exercise routines. (Shown below)

Myopia Exercise Routine	Duration: 25 mins.
Palming	3 minutes
Pumping	3 minutes
Blur Zoning	3 minutes
Acupressure 4	5 minutes
Eye Rolls	2 minutes
Squeeze Blinking	2 minutes
Clock Rotations	2 minutes
Hydrotherapy	5 minutes

Presbyopia/Hyperopia Exercise Routine	Duration: 30 mins.
Palming	3 minutes
Eye Rolls	2 minute
Clock Rotations	2 minute
Squeeze Blinking	1 minute
Pumping	3 minutes
Tromboning	3 minutes
Acupressure 4	5 minutes
Blur Zoning	3 minutes
Shifting	3 minutes
Hydrotherapy	5 minutes

Eye Floaters

Cause:

Eye Floaters (or Spots) are small, cloudy, semi-transparent specks within the vitreous, which is the middle of the eye. Since they are inside your eye, they move when your eyes move, which is why they seem to dart away when you try to look directly at them. Eye Floaters are usually caused by small pieces of protein that was trapped in your eye during birth. They can also be caused by the deterioration of the vitreous fluid (fluid in the middle of the eye), due to aging of the eye. You can usually see Eye Floaters when your eyes are tired or strained.

Exercises:

If you have Eye Floaters, use the exercise routine below. With this exercise routine we are trying to cleanse the eye and stimulate the flow of nutrients.

Exercise Routine	Duration: 25 mins
Palming	3 minutes
Pumping	2 minutes
Slow Blinking	1 minute
Squeeze Blinking	1 minute
Tromboning	2 minutes
Slow Blinking	1 minute
Squeeze Blinking	1 minute
Eye Rolls	2 minutes
Palming	3 minutes
Clock Rotation	2 minutes
Slow Blinking	1 minute
Squeeze Blinking	1 minute
Hydrotherapy	5 minutes

Dry Eye Syndrome (Keratoconjunctivitis Sicca (KCS))

Cause:

Dry Eye Syndrome is an eye condition where there is insufficient tears to nourish the eye properly. Usually caused by poor production of tears or poor drainage. Tears are a necessary part of maintaining the health of the cornea which provides clear vision. They also reduce the risk of eye infection and can wash away foreign bodies from within the eye. There are several factors that can cause Dry Eye Syndrome in people. Below is a list of the most common factors/causes:

- Medications – such as antihistamines, decongestants, antidepressants and blood pressure medications can reduce the production of tears in the eyes.

- Environmental Conditions – such as smoke, dry climates and wind can cause tear evaporation. Also excessive computer work, which causes a person to stare at the screen, can cause drying of the eyes.
- Contact Lens – long term use of contact lens can cause your tear glands to malfunction and tear production decreases. Dry eyes with contacts can also cause a bacterial infection or scratches on the cornea.

Exercises:

Our main goal with this exercise routine is to encourage tear production in the eye. This exercise routine is designed specifically for people with Dry Eye Syndrome.

Exercise Routine	Duration: 25 mins.
Hydrotherapy	3 minutes
Acupressure 1	2 minutes
Slow Blinking	2 minutes
Squeeze Blinking	2 minutes
Acupressure 2	2 minutes
Slow Blinking	2 minutes
Squeeze Blinking	2 minutes
Acupressure 3	2 minutes
Palming	5 minutes
Acupressure 4	3 minutes

Cataract

Cause:

A normal eye consists of the eye's inner lens which is made up of billions of living cells. Sometimes when we get older, these cells start to die which form a Cataract. A Cataract is simply the buildup of cellular debris (or dead cells). Below are some causes of Cataract:

- Ultraviolet light
- Toxic waste products
- Low nutrient levels in the body

Exercises:

Our main focus with this exercise is to boost nutrient levels in the eye, while stimulating and cleansing the debris from the inner lens. If you have Cataracts, along with doing the exercise routine below, we recommend a balanced diet which contains high amounts of Zinc, Vitamin E and Beta-Carotene. For more information on nourishing and cleansing your eyes, see Chapter six.

Exercise Routine	Duration: 25 mins.
Palming	3 minutes
Acupressure 1	2 minutes
Pumping	3 minutes
Acupressure 2	2 minutes
Tromboning	3 minutes
Acupressure 3	2 minutes
Eye Rolls	3 minutes
Acupressure 4	2 minutes
Hydrotherapy	5 minutes

Eyestrain

Cause:

Stress especially on your eyes is an important issue to get fixed. If you do not fix eyestrain, it can seriously deteriorate the performance of your eye and ultimately cause vision problems.

Eyestrain or stress is usually brought on by focusing on something for a long period of time. Now-a-days this eye condition has become increasingly more popular due to the overuse of laptops, TVs, tablets, iPads, or iPhones. Also most jobs require starring at a computer screen all day or reading. The light from the computer screen is causing your eyes to overwork. Especially your retina, which is constantly reflecting light.

This added stress causes symptoms such as:

- Headaches
- Eyelid tics or tension
- Dry eyes
- Bloodshot eyes
- Fatigue
- Loss of concentration
- Blurred or double vision (even with glasses)

Exercises:

If you think you are suffering from eyestrain and have any of the above symptoms, try the exercise routine below:

Exercise Routine	Duration: 25 mins.
Palming	5 minutes
Acupressure 4	5 minutes
Slow Blinking	5 minutes
Hydrotherapy	5 minutes
Palming	5 minutes

NOW TO THE RECOMMENDED EXERCISES

In this section, we'll focus on each of the recommended eye exercises that will help restore your vision and how you can do them. These techniques act like a workout for your eyes – strengthening your eye naturally. Each exercise is useful in helping relief eye stress or strain and help stimulate the flow of nutrients in the eye. Some of the exercises focus on improving your vision through sharpening your eyes ability to see detail, while others work on improving the control of your eye's extraocular muscles.

The exercises don't need a lot of time, and can easily be done throughout the day, without interrupting your daily activities. If you follow this guide and really do the exercises you can gradually improve any common vision problem, regardless of your age or circumstance.

So let's get started!

Pumping

Pumping is used to increase the flow of nutrients while exercising the focusing mechanisms of the eye.

Hold an object 6 inches away from your face. This object can be your finger, a pen, or another small object. *Change focus every two seconds*, between the near object (finger or pen) and a far object at least 15 feet away, such as a tree, billboard, traffic lights etc. Keep changing your focus back and forth between the near object and the far object.

Example: Pen – tree – pen – billboard – pen - truck – pen – traffic light.

Make sure to focus on a new far object each time.

Also make sure your near object is 6 inches away and no farther. Use a ruler to measure the distance of your near object if needed.

Try to briefly focus on a specific detail on both the near and far object before switching.

This exercise can easily be done during TV commercial breaks or office breaks.

If preforming this exercise indoors, you may use an object across the room. Such as a lamp, bookshelf corner or doorframe edge.

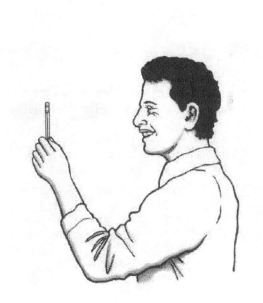

Tromboning

Like Pumping, Tromboning is also used to exercise the focusing mechanisms of the eye and increase the flow of nutrients.

Hold an object at arm's length away from your face. This object can be a finger or pen. ***Breathing slowly and deeply, look at the object*** as you move the object close towards your nose and then stretch your arm back out.

As you inhale, slowly bring the object in towards your face until it touches your nose – make sure to focus on the object. As you exhale, slowly take the object out to arm's length.

Example: inhale – in towards nose, exhale – away from nose.

Make sure to time the movements with your breathing. It's important to have slow, deep breathes, so you aren't moving the object to fast.

When you bring the object close to your nose, you may notice the object going out of focus or forming a double image. Try to keep the object from going out of focus, once you notice it happening, slow down the object and let your eyes focus on a small detail.

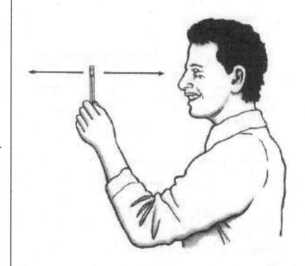

Continue the exercise for as long as possible, keeping the object in full focus the whole time.	

Clock Rotations

Clock Rotations stimulate the flow of nutrients and help control the extraocular muscles around the eye.

Hold an object comfortably at arm's length away from your face. Again this object can be a finger or pen. Now imagine that the object is in the center of clock. 12 o'clock would be directly above it and 3 o'clock would be directly to the right of the object. Keeping your shoulders and neck still, look at the object, and extend your arm all the way up to 12 o'clock. ***Keep looking at the object for 2 -3 seconds. Then return to the center, and repeat this movement 5 times.*** Then move on to 1 o'clock, then 2 o'clock and so on. **Example:** up to 12 o'clock – hold for 3 seconds, repeat x5, up and slightly over to 1 o'clock – hold for 3 seconds, repeat x5, up and slightly over to 2 o'clock – hold for 3 seconds, repeat x5, to the right 3 o'clock – hold for 3 seconds, repeat x5, etc.	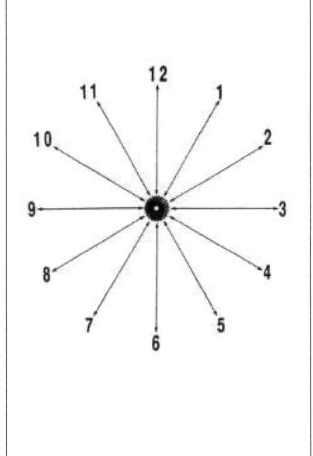

Make sure to stretch the extraocular muscles as far as it will go in each clock position, before moving on to the next position.

It's important to keep the extraocular muscles fully stretched for the full 2- 3 seconds. If you notice a specific clock positon that feels strained, repeat this specific position for another 5 times. Eventually it will become less strained.

Take your time, and slowly move around the clock. Do not rush this exercise. If you stretch the extraocular muscles to hard you will see flashes of light, this means you are stressing the retina.

Eye Rolls

Like Clock Rotations, Eye Rolls also stimulate the flow of nutrients and help control the extraocular muscles around the eye.

Slowly roll your eyes in a complete circle. First clockwise then, counterclockwise. Try to keep the extraocular muscles fully stretched throughout the entire rotation.

Don't look at anything in particular and slowly roll your eyes. We are working on coordination and control, without any jerkiness. If you feel strain or stress in a

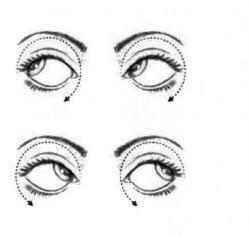

certain location, continue with the eye rolls until it becomes smoother.

Example: eye roll clockwise, eye roll counterclockwise, eye roll clockwise, eye roll counterclockwise, etc.

Take your time, and slowly move around the clock. Do not rush this exercise. If you stretch the extraocular muscles to hard you will see flashes of light, this means you are stressing the retina.

If you are easily motion sick, you may find yourself feeling unwell. Stop, cover your eyes with your hands, and continue the exercise with your eye opens.

Slow Blinking

Slow Blinking is used to reduce visual stress or strain.

Start by breathing deeply and slowly. Once you feel comfortable and relaxed, do a few normal blinks when you inhale for the first time. As you exhale, close your eyes lightly. Exhale slowly allowing your eyes time to rest. When you inhale from now on, keep your eyes open. ***Close your eyes only on exhaling – creating a slow blink.***

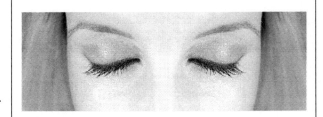

Example: inhale – open eyes, exhale – close eyes, inhale – open eyes, exhale – close eyes, etc.

When you inhale try to completely fill your lungs. When you exhale, slowly push all the air out of your lungs. Repeat this exercise until you feel free of all stress and strain on your body and eyes.

Squeeze Blinking

Squeeze Blinking is used to stimulate the production of tear fluid.

Squeeze you eyelids closed tightly for 3 seconds. Open your eyes wide and do a few normal blinks. Squeeze your eyelids shut again for 3 seconds, then open your eyes again. Continue until your eyes feel moist and relaxed.

Example: squeeze close (hold 3 seconds), open, squeeze close (hold 3 seconds), open, squeeze close (hold 3 seconds), open, etc.

After a couple Squeeze Blinks your eyes will start to create an excess of tear fluid.

Try to isolate your eye muscles when you Squeeze Blink, and not scrunch or wrinkle your forehead or eyebrows.

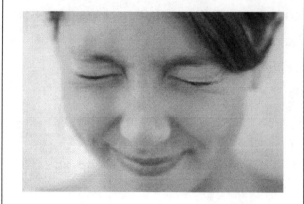

Blur Zoning

Blur Zoning improves the eye's ability to see small details.

Find your Blur Zone in your vision – the spot where you can no longer see an image clear and crisp. Once you have found your Blur Zone, *focus your eyes around the edge of an object, following the major outlines.* Your object can be a tree in the distance if you are nearsighted, or a piece of jewelry held up close if you are farsighted.

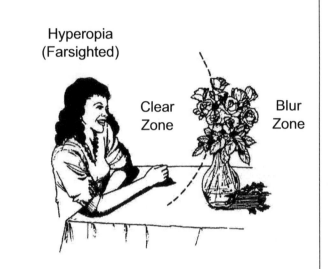

Hyperopia (Farsighted)

Clear Zone

Blur Zone

Go slowly around the object 3 times. Then go around the object again, but this time really study the small details of the object and try to see the exact shape. Do this a couple more times around the object. Then go around the object again 3 times, this time really focusing on the smallest details on the object. If you are nearsighted and are looking at a tree, try to visualize a leaf while looking at a cluster of leaves. If you are farsighted, study a scratch, or metal imperfection on a piece of jewelry. Once you are finished the 3rd time around, rest your eyes.

Example: follow the edge of an object – x3, follow the edge of an object – looking for details x3, then follow the edge of an object – looking for smaller details x3, rest your eyes.

While focusing around the edges of the object, follow the turns and cutouts the outline of the object makes.

Try not to squint to see any of the details. Just stay calm and relaxed and try to visualize smaller and smaller details on the object.

Shifting

Shifting is your eye's natural way of viewing objects. Like Blur Zoning, Shifting improves the eye's ability to see small details.

Using the image on the right as a guideline, focus your eyes on one dot. Now shift or move your focus from that one dot to the next closest dot. Continue doing this until every dot has been shifted to. Then start shifting from one random dot to another random dot on the image. From one corner to the other corner, the middle to the edge, etc.

Now use this method and focus on a real life object, like a house across the street, or bookcase. Don't imagine dots, but focus on specific areas of the object. First start by **shifting from one spot to a closer spot on the object**, then shift from a random spot to another random spot. Do this 3 times on 3

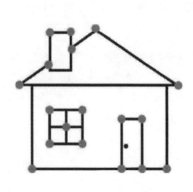

different objects. Once you are finished, make sure to rest your eyes.

Example: Shift from spot to close spot, shift from spot to close spot, shift from spot to random spot, shift from spot to random spot – x3 objects, rest your eyes

Palming

Palming is used to relax your eye muscles and reduce visual stress or strain.

Close your eyes and place your left hand over your left eye, and your right hand over your right eye. You may lay your right fingers on top of your left fingers over your forehead. Rest the heal of your palms on your cheekbones and your elbows on a table. Rest your eyes and relax. Slowly breathing in and out for 30 seconds.

You may want to put a pillow under your elbows for comfort.

Don't press on your eyes, eyelids, or eyebrows. Try to relax all your eye muscles.

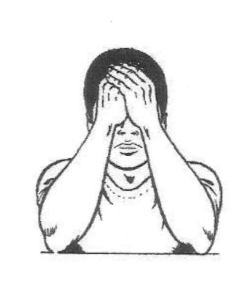

Hydrotherapy

Like Palming, Hydrotherapy is also used to relax your eye muscles and reduce visual stress or strain.

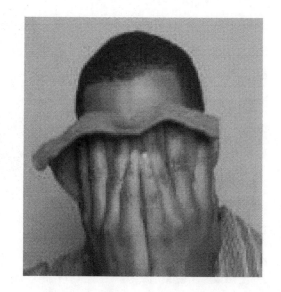

Grab three washcloths and two bowls of water. Fill one bowl with cold water, and fill the other bowl with hot water. Make sure the hot water is hot, but not scalding hot. The cold water should be ice cold. Now dip a washcloth in the hot water, close your eyes and **hold the hot water washcloth against your eyes for 30 seconds.** Now dip another washcloth in the cold water, close your eyes and **hold the cold water washcloth against your eyes for another 30 seconds.** Continue switching between hot and cold washcloths every 30 seconds for 3 – 5 mins. Once you are finished gently massage your closed eyes with the dry washcloth.

Example: hot washcloth – 30 seconds, cold washcloth – 30 seconds, hot washcloth – 30 seconds, cold washcloth – 30 seconds, etc. repeat for 3 – 5 mins, then massage with dry washcloth.

Make sure to rest your eyes muscles and don't push too hard on your eye lids.

Acupressure

Like Palming and Hydrotherapy, Acupressure is also used to relax your eye muscles and reduce visual stress or strain.

1. Upper Eye Socket Close your eyes, place your thumbs on the inside of your upper eye socket, close to your nose, just below your eyebrow. The specific place usually feels like a boney ridge or nub. Once you have found the acupressure location, press firmly with your thumbs for one second, and then release for one second and repeat. Continue this for 30 seconds. **Example:** press, release, press, release, press, release etc.	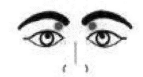
2. Bottom Eye Socket Close your eyes and place your index and middle fingertips on the bottom eye socket bone, right underneath the center of your eye. Press firmly with your two fingers for one second, then release for one second and repeat. Continue this for 30 seconds. **Example:** press, release, press, release, press, release, etc.	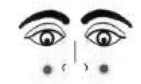
3. Pinching the Bridge of the Nose Close your eyes and place your thumb and pointer finger on either side of the bridge of your nose. Squeeze your finger	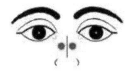

and thumb together for one second, then release for one second, and repeat. Continue this for 30 seconds.

Example: squeeze, release, squeeze, release, squeeze, release, etc.

4. Combine all Acupressure Exercises Together

Combine all the above Acupressure exercises together to give your eyes a thorough massage. Start with Acupressure 1 for 30 seconds, then Acupressure 2 for 30 seconds, then Acupressure 3 for 30 seconds and then using your index and middle finger, gently tab in a circle around your entire eye socket. Start from Acupressure 1 position and work your way out and around the eye. Do this 3 times and then repeat, starting at Acupressure 1 for 30 seconds. Continue this cycle 5 times.

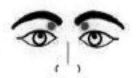

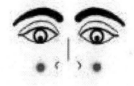

Example: Acupressure 1 – 30 seconds, Acupressure 2 – 30 seconds, Acupressure 3 – 30 seconds, tab around the eye – x3, Acupressure 1 – 30 seconds, Acupressure 2 – 30 seconds, Acupressure 3 – 30 seconds, tab around the eye – x3, etc.

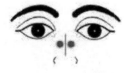

PLEASE REMEMBER TO DO THE RECOMMENDED EXERCISES DAILY FOR OPTIMAL RESULTS

Made in the USA
Las Vegas, NV
30 December 2023

83705623R00015